The Plant-Based Diet

The Most Recent Approach to

a Plant-Based Nutrition to

Lose Weight and Burn Fat

Vegetarian Academy

The information in the following pages is broadly considered a truthful and accurate account of facts and as such, any inattention, use, or misuse of the information in question by the reader will render any resulting actions solely under their purview. There are no scenarios in which the publisher or the original author of this work can be in any fashion deemed liable for any hardship or damages that may befall them after undertaking information described herein.

Additionally, the information in the following pages is intended only for informational purposes and should thus be thought of as universal. As befitting its nature, it is presented without assurance regarding its prolonged validity or interim quality. Trademarks that are mentioned are done without written consent and can in no way be considered an endorsement from the trademark holder.

Tables of Contents

Introduction

Selecting the perfect diet plan can be confusing thanks to the variety of diet plans available these days. Irrespective of what diet plan you opt for, almost all nutritionists and dietitians across the globe recommend diet plans that limit processed foods and that are based more on whole and fresh foods. The Plant-Based Diet is based on these universally preferred foods.

This introduction is going to clear away all ambiguities and doubts regarding the whole-food, plant-based diet plan and provide logical explanations to the benefits it offers.

The whole-food plant-based diet plan is more flexible and understanding than other diets, too. It is mostly comprised of plant-based foods, but you can also have some animal-based products.

Now knowing that eating animal products is a huge risk to your health, it definitely stands as a solid reason why you should opt for plant-based foods. Besides improving your overall health, these foods have numerous benefits to your body. First, they are rich in fiber. Therefore, your digestion will be improved. Their high fiber content, however, demands that dieters should slowly change their usual meals because the bodies take time to adapt. This is a worrying statistic, especially bearing in mind that obesity is linked to cardiovascular diseases and diabetes. Adopting a plant-based diet can help in promoting weight loss. The great thing about this is that you will lose weight naturally without having to worry about gaining again in the future. Usually, the fad diets that people rush to rely on have long-term negative effects. Most people complain about gaining more weight after they had initially shed some pounds. Eating plant foods could prevent such effects. A plant-based diet emphasizes the consumption of anything derived from plants - vegetables, cereals, nuts and seeds - minimizing or excluding animal products. While some may think that a plant-based diet is just another term for a vegetarian or even a vegan diet, there is a fundamental difference. Plant-based diets emphasize the consumption of whole and natural foods and avoid processed foods such as tofu, seitan or packaged products, even if they are technically vegan or vegetarian. A diet composed only of plants will be beneficial in maintaining healthy skin. Providing your skin with the nutrients it requires is the best way of keeping it smooth and glowing. Unfortunately, people lack information about this. As such, they are forced to try different skin products with the hopes of giving their skin a natural glow and clear complexion. Eating right is a solution to almost every disease that we might be suffering from. We have been blinded by the media from realizing that the cure we need is in our food choices.

What is a Plant-based diet?

Though there are variations within a plant-based diet, the major cornerstone of the diet is that plant foods become the central focal point of your diet. This means that you base your meals around food products sourced from plants like vegetables, nuts, seeds, whole grains, fruits, and legumes. Animal products are either cut out completely or are otherwise reduced. How much you reduce your intake of animal products depends upon what you deem best for yourself. However, if you do choose to make animal products such as fish, poultry, meat, dairy, or eggs a part of your diet, they will take a backseat to the plant foods that make up your meals. If this makes you feel nervous, don't worry! This is not a deprivation diet. There are so many appetizing and tasty plant food options out there that you may not even know about! Many of us are so accustomed to meat, animal products and processed foods taking center-stage at meal times that it is hard to imagine what a meal that puts plant foods first would look like. Embarking on a plant-based diet provides you an exciting opportunity to explore new foods and recipes that are not only satisfying and nourishing but are delicious and taste amazing as well.

The following diets all fall under the umbrella of a plant-based diet:

• Vegan: Diet includes vegetables, seeds, nuts, legumes, grains, and fruit and excludes all animal products (i.e. no animal flesh, dairy, or eggs). There are variations within the vegan diet as well such as the fruitarian diet made up mainly of fruits and sometimes nuts and seeds and the raw vegan diet where food is not cooked.

• Vegetarian: Diet includes vegetables, fruit, nuts, legumes, grains, and seeds and excludes meat but may include eggs or dairy. The Ovo-lacto vegetarian diet incorporates dairy and eggs while the Ovo-vegetarian diet incorporates eggs and excludes dairy and the lacto vegetarian diet incorporates dairy but excludes eggs.

• Semi-vegetarianism: Diet is mostly vegetarian but

also incorporates some meat and animal products. The macrobiotic diet is a type of semi-vegetarian diet that emphasizes vegetables, beans, whole grains, naturally processed foods, and may include some seafood, meat, or poultry. The pescatarian diet includes plant foods, eggs, dairy, and seafood but no other types of animal flesh. People who subscribe to a semi-vegetarian diet sometimes describe themselves as flexitarians as well.

The plant-based, whole food diet is really all about trying to only consume whole, unrefined plants. Followers of a plant-based diet like to get their food as organically as possible. If the food is refined, it must only be minimally refined. Vegetables, fruits, whole grains, tubers, and legumes are going to be the most important parts of meals and animal products either take a on a small proportion of the meal or are excluded altogether. This includes meat, dairy products, and eggs. Highly refined products like bleached flour, oil, and refined sugar are usually avoided as well.

Some of these plant-based diets are obviously stricter than others. No one diet is right for everyone, so it is important to understand all the options you have within a plant-based diet so that you can choose which lifestyle is most attractive and feels right to you. Maybe you wantto cut out all animal products and go vegan, consuming only plant foods and products or maybe you prefer keeping some animal products in your diet while making plant foods your main focus. Remember, you are in control of what you eat and what goes into your body. A plant-based diet will likely have more restrictions and parameters than you are used to, so it is crucial that you pick a diet that is not only healthy, but attainable, realistic to adhere to, and enjoyable for you. The plant-based diet is designed to increase your quality of life so it would be counter-productive to choose a diet that makes you feel deprived or unhappy! It is important to set realistic expectations for yourself so that you are able to follow your new diet and are not tempted to stray from it. That being said, following a plant-based diet can be incredibly easy and simple if you follow the right steps and stay committed to your new healthy choices which will not be hard to do once you start feeling the beneficial effects of this health-focused lifestyle.

There has often been some confusion as to whether the

plant based diet is just another word for veganism, or if they are a completely different concept with differentrules, so let's go into that. There are many similarities between the two, but also some distinct differences. Are veganism and a plant based diet the same thing? The short answer is no. Like I said before, the particular diet that is chosen and the label it is given depends on the individual, and the reason they have chosen to live this lifestyle. Many vegans choose to be so because they disagree with the slaughter and poor treatment of farm animals, and so they so not consume these foods. They also usually choose not to use leather, or wear fur or any other animal products. Vegans do not eat any sort of meat, or product containing traces of meat. This includes any broths, or ingredients such as gelatin. Vegans also do not eat any food products that contain ANY ingredient from an animal, including milk or honey. They do not eat any cheese, or yogurt, or margarine or butter, etc. Some slightly more hidden ingredients that contain animal product are whey and casein. These are all avoided. Vegans get most of their food from plant sources, but they are not strictly whole food plant based. They may not be as health conscious, and so many may choose to eat packaged and processed foods yet stay away from those made of animal. This technically still falls within the parameter of their diet.

Plant based folks eat a primarily plant derived diet-as close to nature as possible. But this does not mean that they are vegan, or even vegetarian. They may simply choose to eat mostly fruits, vegetables, nuts and legumes, etc. However, they may still choose to eat meat, and carefully choose meats that are antibiotics free, grass fed, and lived a free-range life. Many plant based dieters believe that meat is still an integral part of a healthy diet, and so they just choose the best quality possible.

Whole food, plant based diets usually take the qualities of both diets, and even go a step further. Keeping foods whole refers to leaving them in their most natural state. So, vegetables and fruit are eaten as they are-fresh, frozen or dried without preservatives or added flavor. Nuts are natural, without salt or sugar; grains are not refined or enriched or bleached. Most foods are prepared at home, or in a restaurant where they chefs share the same standards, as to not degrade any of the ingredients or take away any of their nutritional value. Many processed foods use what is known as plant fragments,rather than whole plants. They are reduced or extracted or otherwise processed in some way. Whatever the specifics of the diet someone chooses, if they tell you that they are vegan or plant based, you should assume that they do not consume any animal products at all, unless they mention it otherwise. This can help you to avoid accidentally serving them something that they will not be willing or able to eat. And feel free to ask someone about their diet, if you are curious. But make sure that they are willing to talk about it, and also that you listen with an open mind-not looking to judge or challenge their decision to adopt that particular diet.

Now, I would like to clarify the way in which I am using the word diet here. I know that many diets are short term and involve cutting calories and foods in order to lose unwanted weight. This is a bit of a touchy thing, because there are many diets out there which can put extreme pressure on the body and will cause weight loss through force or a particular calculation or schedule of eating. This is not what I am referring to in this book. What I will be proposing is that you, the reader, adopt a new addition to your lifestyle that will benefit you, and that you can stick with permanently. This may sound a bit intimidating, to adopt new eating rules for life. However, it is my hope that with my help, you will be able to do this painlessly, and really see benefits from it. You may lose weight; you may have clearer skin and eyes, healthier hair, and even have more abundant energy. And you will help to determine just which benefits you will be rewarded with, by deciding how far you want to go.

The Plant Based Breakfast

Hot Pink Smoothie

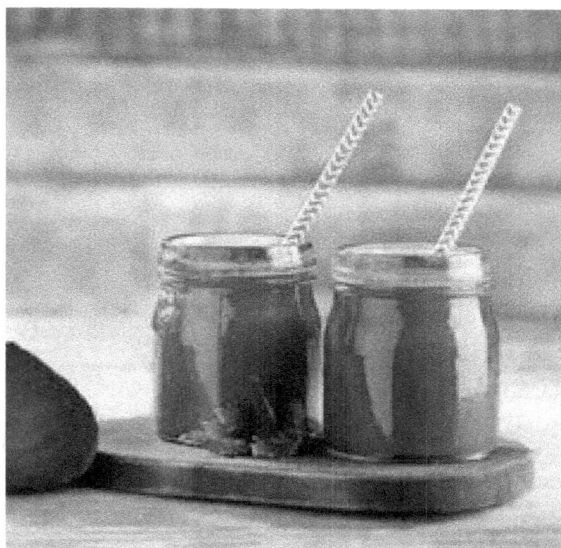

Preparation time: 5 minutes

Cooking time: 0 minute

Servings: 1

Ingredients:

- 1 clementine, peeled, segmented

- 1/2 frozen banana
- 1 small beet, peeled, chopped
- 1/8 teaspoon sea salt
- 1/2 cup raspberries
- 1 tablespoon chia seeds
- 1/4 teaspoon vanilla extract, unsweetened
- 2 tablespoons almond butter
- 1 cup almond milk, unsweetened

Method:

1. Place all the ingredients in the order in a food processor or blender and then pulse for 2 to 3 minutes at high speed until smooth.
2. Pour the smoothie into a glass and then serve.

Nutrition Value:

- Calories: 278 Cal
- Fat: 5.6 g
- Carbs: 37.2 g
- Protein: 6.2 g
- Fiber: 13.2 g

Maca Caramel Frap

Preparation time: 5 minutes

Cooking time: 0 minute

Servings: 4

Ingredients:

- 1/2 of frozen banana, sliced
- 1/4 cup cashews, soaked for 4 hours
- 2 Medjool dates, pitted
- 1 teaspoon maca powder
- 1/8 teaspoon sea salt
- 1/2 teaspoon vanilla extract, unsweetened
- 1/4 cup almond milk, unsweetened
- 1/4 cup cold coffee, brewed

Method:

Place all the ingredients in the order in a food processor or blender and then pulse for 2 to 3 minutes at high speed until smooth.

Pour the smoothie into a glass and then serve.

Nutrition Value:

- Calories: 450 Cal
- Fat: 170 g
- Carbs: 64 g
- Protein: 7 g
- Fiber: 0 g

Peanut Butter Vanilla Green Shake

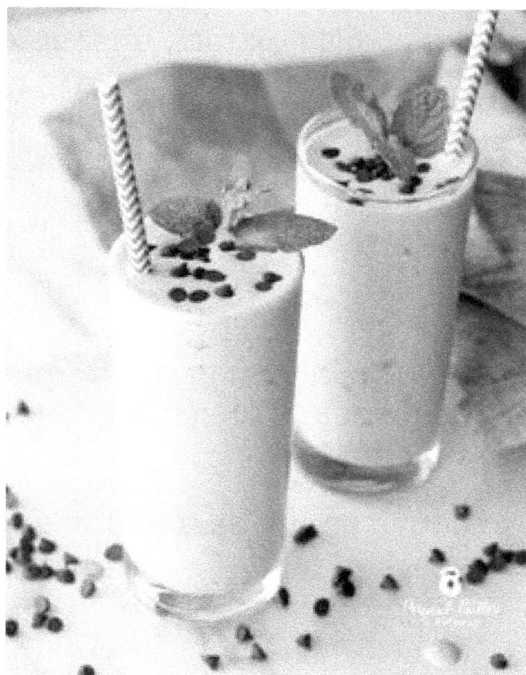

Preparation time: 5 minutes

Cooking time: 0 minute

Servings: 1

Ingredients:

- 1 teaspoon flax seeds
- 1 frozen banana

- 1 cup baby spinach
- 1/8 teaspoon sea salt
- 1/2 teaspoon ground cinnamon
- 1/4 teaspoon vanilla extract, unsweetened
- 2 tablespoons peanut butter, unsweetened
- 1/4 cup ice
- 1 cup coconut milk, unsweetened

Method:

Place all the ingredients in the order in a food processor or blender and then pulse for 2 to 3 minutes at high speed until smooth.

Pour the smoothie into a glass and then serve.

Nutrition Value:

- Calories: 298 Cal
- Fat: 11 g
- Carbs: 32 g
- Protein: 24 g
- Fiber: 8 g

Green Colada

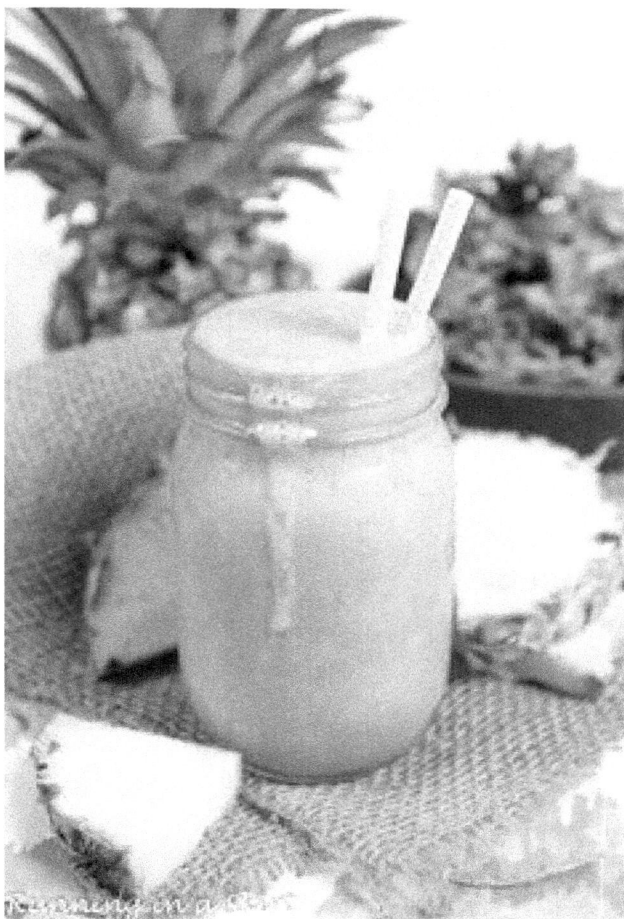

Preparation time: 5 minutes

Cooking time: 0 minute

Servings: 1

Ingredients:

- 1/2 cup frozen pineapple chunks
- 1/2 banana
- 1/2 teaspoon spirulina powder
- 1/4 teaspoon vanilla extract, unsweetened
- 1 cup of coconut milk

Method:

1. Place all the ingredients in the order in a food processor or blender and then pulse for 2 to 3 minutes at high speed until smooth.
2. Pour the smoothie into a glass and then serve.

Nutrition Value:

- Calories: 127 Cal
- Fat: 3 g
- Carbs: 25 g
- Protein: 3 g
- Fiber: 4 g

Chocolate Oat Smoothie

Preparation time: 5 minutes

Cooking time: 0 minute

Servings: 1

Ingredients:

- ¼ cup rolled oats
- 1 ½ tablespoon cocoa powder, unsweetened
- 1 teaspoon flax seeds
- 1 large frozen banana
- 1/8 teaspoon sea salt
- 1/8 teaspoon cinnamon
- ¼ teaspoon vanilla extract, unsweetened
- 2 tablespoons almond butter
- 1 cup coconut milk, unsweetened

Method:

1. Place all the ingredients in the order in a food processor or blender and then pulse for 2 to 3 minutes at high speed until smooth.

2. Pour the smoothie into a glass and then serve.

Nutrition Value:

Calories: 262 Cal

Fat: 7.3 g

Carbs: 50.4 g

Protein: 8.1 g

Fiber: 9.6 g

Peach Crumble Shake

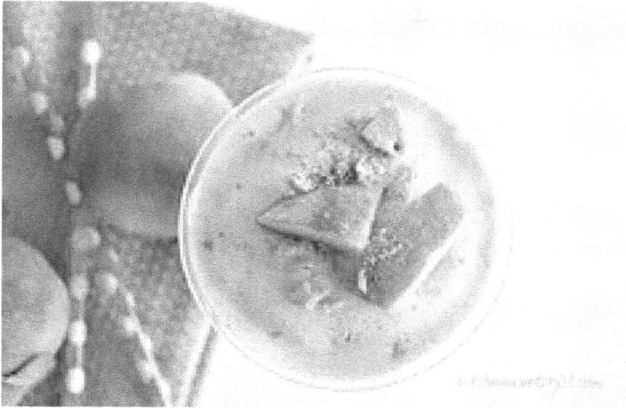

Preparation time: 5 minutes

Cooking time: 0 minute

Servings: 1

Ingredients:

- 1 tablespoon chia seeds
- ¼ cup rolled oats
- 2 peaches, pitted, sliced
- ¾ teaspoon ground cinnamon
- 1 Medjool date, pitted
- ½ teaspoon vanilla extract, unsweetened
- 2 tablespoons lemon juice

- ½ cup of water
- 1 tablespoon coconut butter
- 1 cup coconut milk, unsweetened

Method:

1. Place all the ingredients in the order in a food processor or blender and then pulse for 2 to 3 minutes at high speed until smooth.

2. Pour the smoothie into a glass and then serve.

Nutrition Value:

- Calories: 270 Cal
- Fat: 4 g
- Carbs: 28 g
- Protein: 25 g
- Fiber: 3 g

Wild Ginger Green Smoothie

Preparation time: 5 minutes

Cooking time: 0 minute

Servings: 1

Ingredients:

- 1/2 cup pineapple chunks, frozen
- 1/2 cup chopped kale
- 1/2 frozen banana
- 1 tablespoon lime juice
- 2 inches ginger, peeled, chopped
- 1/2 cup coconut milk, unsweetened
- 1/2 cup coconut water

Method:

1. Place all the ingredients in the order in a food processor or blender and then pulse for 2 to 3 minutes at high speed until smooth.
2. Pour the smoothie into a glass and then serve.

Nutrition Value:

- Calories: 331 Cal
- Fat: 14 g
- Carbs: 40 g
- Protein: 16 g
- Fiber: 9 g

Berry Beet Velvet Smoothie

Preparation time: 5 minutes

Cooking time: 0 minute

Servings: 1

Ingredients:

- 1/2 of frozen banana
- 1 cup mixed red berries
- 1 Medjool date, pitted
- 1 small beet, peeled, chopped
- 1 tablespoon cacao powder
- 1 teaspoon chia seeds
- 1/4 teaspoon vanilla extract, unsweetened
- 1/2 teaspoon lemon juice
- 2 teaspoons coconut butter
- 1 cup coconut milk, unsweetened

Method:

1. Place all the ingredients in the order in a food processor or blender and then pulse for 2 to 3

minutes at high speed until smooth.

2. Pour the smoothie into a glass and then serve.

Nutrition Value:

- Calories: 234 Cal
- Fat: 5 g
- Carbs: 42 g
- Protein: 11 g
- Fiber: 7 g

Spiced Strawberry Smoothie

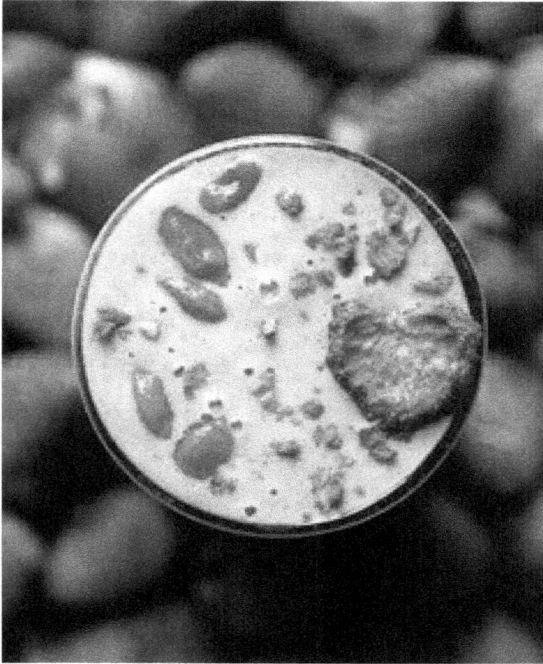

Preparation time: 5 minutes

Cooking time: 0 minute

Servings: 1

Ingredients:

- 1 tablespoon goji berries, soaked
- 1 cup strawberries

- 1/8 teaspoon sea salt
- 1 frozen banana
- 1 Medjool date, pitted
- 1 scoop vanilla-flavored whey protein
- 2 tablespoons lemon juice
- ¼ teaspoon ground ginger
- ½ teaspoon ground cinnamon
- 1 tablespoon almond butter
- 1 cup almond milk, unsweetened

Method:

1. Place all the ingredients in the order in a food processor or blender and then pulse for 2 to 3 minutes at high speed until smooth.
2. Pour the smoothie into a glass and then serve.

Nutrition Value:

- Calories: 182 Cal
- Fat: 1.3 g
- Carbs: 34 g
- Protein: 6.4 g
- Fiber: 0.7 g

Banana Bread Shake With Walnut Milk

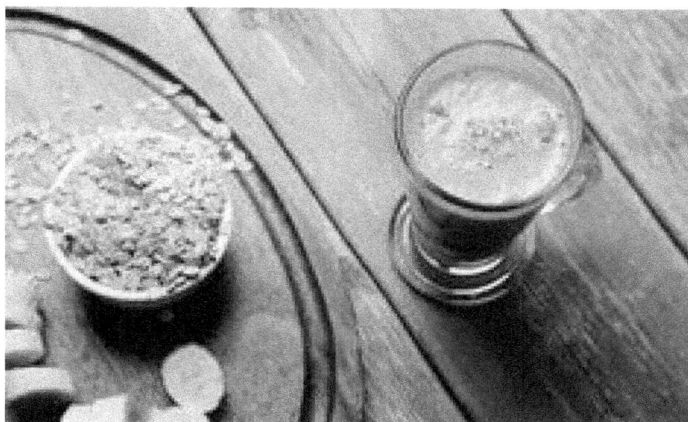

Preparation time: 5 minutes

Cooking time: 0 minute

Servings: 2

Ingredients:

- 2 cups sliced frozen bananas
- 3 cups walnut milk
- 1/8 teaspoon grated nutmeg
- 1 tablespoon maple syrup
- 1 teaspoon ground cinnamon

- 1/2 teaspoon vanilla extract, unsweetened
- 2 tablespoons cacao nibs

Method:

1. Place all the ingredients in the order in a food processor or blender and then pulse for 2 to 3 minutes at high speed until smooth.
2. Pour the smoothie into two glasses and then serve.
3.

Nutrition Value:

Calories: 339.8 Cal

Fat: 19 g

Carbs: 39 g

Protein: 4.3 g

Fiber: 1 g

Double Chocolate Hazelnut Espresso Shake

Preparation time: 5 minutes

Cooking time: 0 minute

Servings: 1

Ingredients:

- 1 frozen banana, sliced
- 1/4 cup roasted hazelnuts
- 4 Medjool dates, pitted, soaked
- 2 tablespoons cacao nibs, unsweetened
- 1 1/2 tablespoons cacao powder, unsweetened
- 1/8 teaspoon sea salt
- 1 teaspoon vanilla extract, unsweetened
- 1 cup almond milk, unsweetened
- 1/2 cup ice
- 4 ounces espresso, chilled

Method:

1. Place all the ingredients in the order in a food

processor or blender and then pulse for 2 to 3 minutes at high speed until smooth.

2. Pour the smoothie into a glass and then serve.

Nutrition Value:

- Calories: 210 Cal
- Fat: 5 g
- Carbs: 27 g
- Protein: 16.8 g
- Fiber: 0.2 g

Strawberry, Banana and Coconut Shake

Preparation time: 5 minutes

Cooking time: 0 minute

Servings: 1

Ingredients:

- 1 tablespoon coconut flakes
- 1 1/2 cups frozen banana slices
- 8 strawberries, sliced
- 1/2 cup coconut milk, unsweetened
- 1/4 cup strawberries for topping

Method:

1. Place all the ingredients in the order in a food processor or blender, except for topping and then pulse for 2 to 3 minutes at high speed until smooth.
2. Pour the smoothie into a glass and then serve.

Nutrition Value:

- Calories: 335 Cal
- Fat: 5 g
- Carbs: 75 g
- Protein: 4 g
- Fiber: 9 g

Tropical Vibes Green Smoothie

Preparation time: 5 minutes

Cooking time: 0 minute

Servings: 1

Ingredients:

- 2 stalks of kale, ripped
- 1 frozen banana
- 1 mango, peeled, pitted, chopped
- 1/8 teaspoon sea salt
- ¼ cup of coconut yogurt
- ½ teaspoon vanilla extract, unsweetened
- 1 tablespoon ginger juice
- ½ cup of orange juice
- ½ cup of coconut water

Method:

1. Place all the ingredients in the order in a food processor or blender and then pulse for 2 to 3 minutes at high speed until smooth.
2. Pour the smoothie into a glass and then serve.

Nutrition Value:

- Calories: 197.5 Cal
- Fat: 1.3 g
- Carbs: 30 g
- Protein: 16.3 g
- Fiber: 4.8 g

Peanut Butter and Mocha Smoothie

Preparation time: 5 minutes

Cooking time: 0 minute

Servings: 1

Ingredients:

- 1 frozen banana, chopped
- 1 scoop of chocolate protein powder
- 2 tablespoons rolled oats
- 1/8 teaspoon sea salt
- ¼ teaspoon vanilla extract, unsweetened
- 1 teaspoon cocoa powder, unsweetened
- 2 tablespoons peanut butter
- 1 shot of espresso
- ½ cup almond milk, unsweetened

Method:

1. Place all the ingredients in the order in a food processor or blender and then pulse for 2 to 3 minutes at high speed until smooth.

2. Pour the smoothie into a glass and then serve.

Nutrition Value:

- Calories: 380 Cal
- Fat: 14 g
- Carbs: 29 g
- Protein: 38 g
- Fiber: 4 g

Tahini Shake with Cinnamon and Lime

Preparation time: 5 minutes

Cooking time: 0 minute

Servings: 1

Ingredients:

- 1 frozen banana
- 2 tablespoons tahini
- 1/8 teaspoon sea salt
- ¾ teaspoon ground cinnamon
- ¼ teaspoon vanilla extract, unsweetened
- 2 teaspoons lime juice
- 1 cup almond milk, unsweetened

Method:

1. Place all the ingredients in the order in a food processor or blender and then pulse for 2 to 3 minutes at high speed until smooth.
2. Pour the smoothie into a glass and then serve.

Nutrition Value:

- Calories: 225 Cal
- Fat: 15 g
- Carbs: 22 g
- Protein: 6 g
- Fiber: 8 g

The Plant Based Lunch

Grilled Eggplant Roll-Ups

Preparation Time: 5 min

Cooking Time: 8 min

servings: 8

Ingredients:

- Olive oil, two tablespoons
- Basil, fresh, chopped, two tablespoons
- Onion, one half sliced paper-thin
- Bell pepper, one half sliced paper-thin
- Tomato, one large
- Eggplant, one medium

Method:

After cutting off both of the ends of the eggplant, slice it into strips the long way that is about a quarter-inch thick. Slice the onion, bell pepper, and the tomato very thinly and set to the side. Brush the olive oil onto the slices of eggplant and grill them in a skillet for three minutes on each side. When both sides are grilled, lay the slices of eggplant on a plate and lay a slice each of tomato, onion, and bell pepper on each zucchini slice. Sprinkle all with the black pepper and the basil. Carefully roll each slice as far as it will roll.

Nutrition:

- Calorie 59
- 4 grams carbs
- 3 grams protein
- 3 grams fat

Veggie Stuffed Peppers

Preparation Time: 30 min

servings: 6

Ingredients:

- Balsamic vinegar, two tablespoons
- Parsley, fresh, one-quarter cup chopped
- Scallions, one bunch, cleaned and sliced
- Cucumber, one half, peeled and diced
- Celery, washed and diced four stalks
- Cherry tomatoes cut in quarters, one cup
- Green bell peppers, three, cleaned and cut in half across the middle
- Salt, one half teaspoon
- Dijon mustard, three tablespoons
- Black pepper, one teaspoon

Method:

In one bowl, mix together the mustard, rice wine vinegar, salt, and pepper. Add in the tomatoes, cucumbers, scallions, and celery and mix gently but well. Use a spoon to stuff this mix into the pepper halves.

Nutrition:

- Calories 117
- 9 grams carbs
- 7 grams protein
- 3 grams fat

Sprout Wraps

Preparation Time: 15 min

servings: 2

Ingredients:

- Tortillas, whole-wheat , two large
- Parsley, one-half cup chopped
- Onion, green, two stalks
- Black pepper, one teaspoon
- Cucumber, one sliced thin
- Bean sprouts, one cup
- Salt, one half teaspoon
- Lemon juice, one tablespoon
- Olive oil, one tablespoon

Method:

Lay out each of the tortilla wraps on a plate. Divide evenly all of the ingredients between the two tortillas, leaving about two inches on either side for rolling the tortilla up. When you have added all of the ingredients on the tortilla, then fold in the sides and roll the tortilla up into a cylinder shape.

Nutrition:

- Calories 226
- 12 grams carbs
- 10 grams protein
- 3 grams fat

Collard Wraps

Preparation Time: 20 min

servings: 4

Ingredients:

- Wrap
- Cherry tomatoes, four cut in half
- Black olives, sliced, one quarter cup
- Purple onion, one-half cup diced fine
- Red bell pepper, one half of one cut in julienne strips
- Cucumber, one medium-sized cut in julienne strips
- Green collard leaves, four large
- Sauce
- Black pepper, one teaspoon
- Salt, one half teaspoon
- Dill, fresh, minced, two tablespoons
- Cucumber, seeded and grated, one quarter cup
- Olive oil, two tablespoons
- White vinegar, one tablespoon

- Garlic powder, one teaspoon

Method:

Place all of the ingredients on the list for the sauce in a mixing bowl and mix well. Store the dressing in the refrigerator. Wash off the collard leaves and dry them and then cut off the stem from each leaf. Cover each leaf with two tablespoons of the sauce you just made. In the middle of the collard leaf layer, all of the other ingredients. Fold the leaf up like a burrito by first folding the ends in and then rolling the leaf until it is all rolled. Cut into slices and serve with more dressing for dipping.

Nutrition per wrap:

- Calories 165, 7.36
- grams carbs, 6.98
- grams protein, 11.25
- grams fat

Grape Tomatoes and Spiral Zucchini

Preparation Time: 5 min

Cooking Time: 10 min

servings: 2

Ingredients:

- Zucchini, one large cut in spirals
- Basil, fresh, chopped, one tablespoon
- Black pepper, one teaspoon
- Rosemary, one teaspoon
- Salt, one half teaspoon
- Lemon juice, one tablespoon
- Crushed red pepper flakes, one quarter teaspoon
- Grape tomatoes, one cup cut in half
- Garlic, minced, two tablespoons
- Olive oil, one tablespoon

Method:

Fry the minced garlic in the olive oil for one minute. Pour

in the pepper, salt, red pepper flakes, and the tomatoes and mix well, then turn the heat lower. Simmer this mix for fifteen minutes. Add in the basil, rosemary, and the zucchini spiral noodles and turn the heat back up and Cooking Time: for two minutes, stirring constantly. Drizzle the lemon juice over all of it and serve.

Nutrition:

- Calories 117
- grams carbs: 13
- grams protein: 4
- grams fat: 5

Cauliflower Fried Rice

Preparation Time: 5 min

Cooking Time: 10 min

servings: 4

Ingredients:

- Riced cauliflower, twelve ounces frozen or fresh
- Sesame oil, one tablespoon
- Soy sauce, two tablespoons
- Carrot, one-quarter cup chopped fine
- Tofu, firm, cut into crumbles
- Garlic, minced, two tablespoons
- Green onion, one quarter cup

Method:

Cooking Time: the carrots and the riced cauliflower in the sesame oil for about five minutes, stirring sometimes. Stir in this mix the chopped green onion and the garlic and Cooking Time: for one minute. Add the tofu to the rice mix and stir about two to three minutes. Just before serving mix in the soy sauce.

Nutrition:

- 114 Calories
- carbs 6g
- protein: 4g
- fat 8g

Mediterranean Style Pasta

Preparation Time: 10 min

Cooking Time: 15 min

servings: 4

Ingredients:

- Whole-wheat pasta, twelve ounces cooked
- Nutritional yeast, one quarter cup
- Kalamata olives, ten, cut in half
- Parsley, chopped, two tablespoons
- Capers, two tablespoons
- Tomatoes, diced, one half cup
- Salt, one half teaspoon
- Black pepper, one teaspoon
- Garlic, minced, two tablespoons
- Olive oil, two tablespoons
- Spinach, one cup, packed

Method:

Fry together in the olive oil, the salt, spinach, and the pepper for ten minutes until the spinach wilts. Add in the capers, parsley, olives, and tomatoes and mix well, cooking for another five minutes. Blend in the whole-wheat pasta, sprinkle on the nutritional yeast, and serve immediately.

Nutrition:

- Calories 231,
- 6.5 grams carbs, ,
- 6.5 grams protein,
- 20 grams fat

Squash and Sweet Potato Patties

Preparation Time: 15 minutes

Cooking Time: 10 minutes

servings: 2

Ingredients:

- Olive oil, two tablespoons
- Salt, one half teaspoon
- Black pepper, one teaspoon
- Parsley, dried, one quarter teaspoon
- Cumin, ground, one quarter teaspoon
- Garlic powder, one half teaspoon
- Sweet potato, cooked and mashed, two cups
- Squash, shredded, one cup

Method:

Mix the sweet potato and squash in a mixing bowl. Add in all of the spices and mix these ingredients well. Heat the oil in a skillet and separate the mix into four equal portions. Drop the portions into the oil and flatten slightly with a fork. Fry each of the patties for five minutes on each side and serve.

Nutrition per patty:

- Calories 112
- 6 grams carbs
- 3 grams protein
- 9 grams fat

Stuffed Artichokes

Preparation Time: 45 min

Cooking Time: 30 min

servings: 6

Ingredients:

- Artichokes, three
- Celery salt, one half teaspoon
- Mushroom, chopped, one half cup
- Salt, one half teaspoon
- Black pepper, one teaspoon
- Onion, minced, two tablespoons
- Lemon juice, two tablespoons
- Parsley, chopped, one tablespoon

Method:

Heat oven to 375. Tear off and discard the outside leaves of the artichokes. Cut the inside of the artichokes in half across the middle. Drop the halves into already boiling water and Cooking Time: them for twenty minutes. Mix together the seasonings, onions, mushrooms, lemon juice, chili sauce, and parsley and spoon this mixture into the boiled artichoke hearts. Place the filled hearts into a baking pan and bake for thirty minutes.

Nutrition:

- Calories 425
- 17 grams carbs
- 18 grams protein
- 21 grams fat

Lima Bean Casserole

Preparation Time: 15 min

Cooking Time: 30 min

servings: 5

Ingredients:

- Lima beans, canned two cups
- Lemon juice, two teaspoons
- Thyme, one half teaspoon
- Black pepper, one teaspoon
- Nutritional yeast, one half cup
- Olive oil, two tablespoons
- Dry mustard, two teaspoons
- Salt, one half teaspoon
- Cumin, one teaspoon

Method:

Heat oven to 375. Drain the beans and save the liquid. Dump the drained beans into an eight by eight-inch baking pan. Add the olive oil with the bean liquid to a skillet and heat until the warm. Add in the pepper, salt, cumin, thyme, dry mustard, and lemon juice and stir together well. Pour this mix over the beans in the baking pan and cover with the nutritional yeast. Bake for thirty minutes.

Nutrition:

- Calories 194,
- 19 grams carbs,
- 6 grams protein,
- 7 grams fat

Corn and Okra Casserole

Preparation Time: 20 min

Cooking Time: 30 min

servings: 6

Ingredients:

- Okra, one pound
- Garlic, one clove sliced
- Parsley, chopped, one tablespoon
- Olive oil, three tablespoons
- Tomatoes, two large diced
- Green bell pepper, one cleaned and sliced
- Corn, whole kernel, one can
- Onion, one small, sliced

Method:

Heat oven to 375. Cut the okra into bite-sized chunks. Cooking Time: the garlic, onion, okra, and green pepper in the olive oil for ten minutes. Stir in the parsley and the tomatoes and Cooking Time: for an additional ten minutes. Pour in the corn and dump the entire mixture into a nine by nine-inch baking pan and bake, not covered, for thirty minutes.

Nutrition:

- Calories 125
- 17 grams carbs
- 4 grams protein
- 2 grams fat

Cucumber Tomato Toast

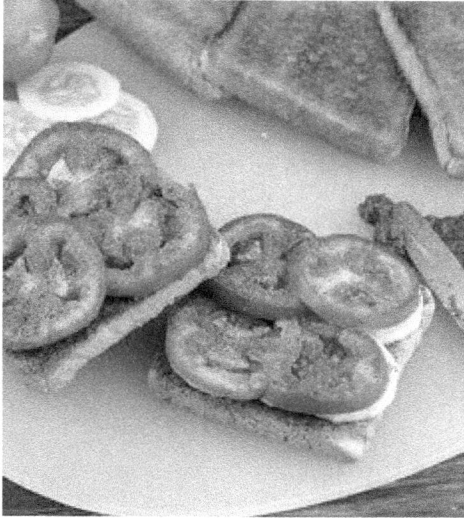

Preparation Time: 5 min

servings: 1

Ingredients:

- Balsamic vinegar, one teaspoon
- Oregano, dried, one half teaspoon
- Cucumber, one half diced
- Tomato, one half diced
- Whole-grain flatbread, two slices
- Salt one half teaspoon

- Thyme, one quarter teaspoon
- Black pepper, one half teaspoon
- Olive oil, one teaspoon

Method:

Mix well the pepper, salt, olive oil, oregano, thyme, dill, tomato, and cucumber. Top the flatbread with the mix. Drizzle on vinegar to taste.

Nutrition info:

- Calories 177
- 8 grams fat
- 24 grams carbs
- 3 grams protein

Pasta Pomodoro with Olives and White Beans

Preparation Time: 30 minutes

servings: 2

Ingredients:

- Ziti or rigatoni, whole-wheat , four ounces
- Nutritional yeast, one half cup
- Cannellini beans, one fifteen ounce can drain and rinse
- Black pepper, one half teaspoon
- Basil, ground, one quarter cup
- Black olives, two tablespoons chopped
- Tomatoes, two medium-sized diced
- Garlic, minced, two tablespoons
- Olive oil, one tablespoon

Method:

Cooking Time: the pasta per the package instructions. Cooking Time: the beans and garlic in the hot oil for five minutes. Take the pan from the heat. Add in the olives, pepper, basil, and tomatoes and mix well. Place the pasta on two plates, evenly divided and top with the tomato bean mix. Sprinkle on the nutritional yeast and serve.

Nutrition info:

- Calories 478
- 16 grams fat
- 14 grams fiber
- 74 grams carbs
- 21 grams protein

Bean Bolognese

Preparation Time: 40 minutes

servings: 4

Ingredients:

- White beans, one fourteen ounce can drain and rinse
- Fettuccini, whole-wheat , eight ounces
- Onion, one small chop
- Olive oil, two tablespoons
- Parsley, fresh, chopped, one-quarter cup divided
- Tomatoes, diced, one fourteen ounce can
- Balsamic vinegar, one half cup
- Celery, one quarter cup chop
- Carrot, one half cup chop
- Bay leaf, one
- Garlic, minced, two tablespoons
- Salt, one half teaspoon

Method:

Cooking Time: the pasta per the package directions.

Cooking Time: carrot, onion, celery, and garlic in the oil for ten minutes. Add in the bay leaf and salt and stir for one minute. Throw away the bay leaf. Pour in the balsamic vinegar and boil for five minutes. Add in the beans, tomatoes, and two tablespoons of the parsley to the skillet and simmer for five minutes, stirring often. Spoon the pasta into four bowls. Top the pasta with the sauce mix from the skillet. Sprinkle on the remainder of the parsley and serve.

Nutrition info:

- Calories 442
- 11 grams fat
- 13 grams fiber
- 68 grams carbs
- 18 grams protein

Fusilli with Tomatoes and Squash

Preparation Time: 25 minutes

servings: 6

Ingredients:

- Fusilli pasta, twelve ounces
- Grape tomatoes, two cups, sliced in half
- Black pepper, one half teaspoon
- Rosemary, one half teaspoon
- Squash, yellow, one pound
- Onion, yellow, one thin slice
- Salt, one half teaspoon
- Thyme, chop, one tablespoon
- Olive oil, two tablespoons

Method:

Cooking Time: the pasta per the package directions. Cut the neck off the squash. Cut the squash into quarters longwise and slice thin. Cooking Time: onion, pepper, squash, thyme, and salt in the hot olive oil for ten minutes, stirring often. Pour in the tomatoes and Cooking

Time: for five more minutes. Add in the cooked pasta and mix well.

Nutrition info:

- Calories 311
- 9 grams fat
- 4 grams fiber
- 49 grams carbs
- 10 grams proteins

The Plant Based Dinner

Farro and Veggies

Preparation Time: 15 minutes

Cooking Time: 40 minutes

servings: 4

Ingredients:

- Farro and Veggies
- Farro, two cups cooked
- Olive oil, two tablespoons
- Red bell pepper, one diced
- Butter lettuce, one head, torn
- Balsamic vinegar, two tablespoons
- Dill, dried, one tablespoon
- Black pepper, one teaspoon
- Rosemary, one teaspoon
- Salt, one half teaspoon
- Red potatoes, one pound cut in wedges
- Oregano, dried, one tablespoon

- Paprika, one tablespoon
- Garlic, minced, two tablespoons
- Butter lettuce, one head torn
- Red onion, cucumber, green and/or black olives for serving
- Red Wine Vinaigrette
- Olive oil, one quarter cup
- Balsamic vinegar, three tablespoons
- Lemon juice, two tablespoons
- Oregano, dried, one tablespoon
- Garlic, minced, one tablespoon
- Red pepper flakes, crushed, one quarter teaspoon
- Salt, one half teaspoon
- Black pepper, one teaspoon

Method:

Heat oven to 425. Mix together well the garlic, paprika, rosemary, salt, pepper, oregano, dill, balsamic vinegar, and one tablespoon of the olive oil. Lay the bell peppers and potatoes in a nine by thirteen-inch baking dish and cover with the seasoning mixture you just assembled. Bake the veggies for forty-five minutes. While the veggies are baking blend together well all the vinaigrette ingredients. Divide the lettuce between four bowls and cover with the farro and add the roasted veggie mix. Drizzle the vinaigrette over the mix in the bowls and serve with olives, onion, and cucumber on the side.

Nutrition info:

- Calories 782
- grams fat 3.8
- 19 grams carbs
- 4.2 grams fiber

Stuffed Eggplant

Preparation Time: 10 min

Cooking Time: 40 min

servings: 4

Ingredients:

- Eggplant, two medium-size cut in half
- Quinoa, cooked, two cups
- Mushrooms, button, one cup thin-slice
- Red onion, one diced
- Parsley, chopped fresh, three tablespoons for garnish
- Salt, one half teaspoon
- Black pepper, one teaspoon
- Turmeric, one teaspoon
- Thyme, dried, one tablespoon
- Kale, two cups chopped
- Lemon juice, one tablespoon
- Lemon zest, one tablespoon
- Garlic, powdered, one tablespoon
- Olive oil, three tablespoons divided

Method:

Heat oven to 400. Use a spoon to scoop one-third of the eggplant flesh out; save it for another use. Use half of the olive oil to coat the halves of the eggplant and place them on a parchment paper-covered baking pan with the inside facing up. Use the rest of the olive oil for cooking the kale, garlic, mushrooms, onions, and quinoa for five minutes. Use lemon juice, lemon zest, pepper, salt, and thyme to season this mix. Use the mix to fill the eggplant halves and bake for twenty minutes. Sprinkle with parsley serve.

Nutrition info:

- Calories 339
- 15 grams fat
- 46 grams carbs
- 12 grams protein

Veggie Rice Skillet

Preparation Time: 15 min

Cooking Time: 25 min

servings: four to six

Serve as dinner and take the leftovers to lunch the next day

Ingredients:

- Parsley, fresh chopped, one third cup
- Green olives, one cup
- Vegetable broth, two and one half cups
- Garlic, minced, two tablespoons
- Olive oil, two tablespoons
- Rosemary, one teaspoon
- Marjoram, one teaspoon
- Salt, one half teaspoon
- Black pepper, one teaspoon
- Oregano, dried, one teaspoon
- Rice, brown or wild, one cup
- Red onion, one half minced
- Lemons, three

Method:

Add the onion and garlic to the olive oil and fry for five minutes. Pour in the broth, rice, and veggies and mix well and let this mixture boil. Let this simmer over a lowered heat for twenty to twenty-five minutes, or until the rice is cooked. Top the individual servings with fresh parsley, olives, and lemon slices.

Nutrition info

- Calories 903
- 55 grams fat
- 54 grams carbs
- 48 grams protein

Brown Rice and Mushroom Risotto

Preparation Time: 20 minutes

Cooking Time: 25 minutes

servings: 6

Ingredients:

- Black pepper, one teaspoon
- Salt, one half teaspoon
- Parsley, dried, one tablespoon
- Brown rice, four cups
- Vegetable broth, two cups divided
- Mushrooms, button, one cup, sliced thin
- Shallot, one large, minced
- Onion, one small, well diced
- Garlic, minced, two tablespoons
- Marjoram, one teaspoon
- Olive oil, two tablespoons

Method:

Fry the shallot, onion, and garlic in the olive oil for five minutes. Pour in one cup of the vegetable's broth and the mushrooms, Cooking Time: for five more minutes. Into this mixture, add the other cup of the vegetable broth and the brown rice, cooking for ten minutes while stirring often. Pour in the salt, pepper, and parsley and turn the heat under the pot to low . Simmer this mixture for ten to fifteen minutes or until the rice is completely cooked.

Nutrition:

- Calories 297
- 7.5 grams carbs
- 7 grams protein
- 26 grams fat

Roast Baby Eggplant

Preparation Time: 20 min

Cooking Time: 45 min

servings: 4

Ingredients:

- To Cooking Time:
- Baby eggplant, eight
- Black pepper, one teaspoon
- Olive oil, two tablespoons
- Salt, one teaspoon
- For Serving
- Salt, one teaspoon
- Olive oil, two tablespoons
- Black pepper, one teaspoon
- Nutritional yeast, one half cup

Method:

Heat oven to 350. Wipe off the eggplants and cut each one in half down the long way. Lay them on a baking pan with the inside up and coat the insides with olive oil and sprinkle on pepper and salt. Bake the baby eggplant for forty-five minutes or until they become soft and brown slightly. Just before you serve them, top each eggplant half with a teaspoon of the nutritional yeast and top that with the olive oil, pepper, and salt.

Nutrition per half an eggplant:

- Calories 44
- 1 gram carbs
- 1 gram protein
- 4 grams fat

Mediterranean Style Spaghetti Squash

Preparation Time: 20 min

servings: 2

Ingredients:

- Baked spaghetti squash, two cups
- Red onion, thin slice, one quarter cup
- Olive oil, two tablespoons
- Salt, one half teaspoon
- Baby spinach, torn, one cup
- Cherry tomatoes, six, cut in half
- Garlic, minced, one teaspoon
- Thyme, dried, one teaspoon
- Rosemary, one teaspoon
- Marjoram, one teaspoon
- Chickpeas, one-third cup, rinse and drain
- Parsley, fresh, chopped, one half cup

Method:

Fry the onion and the garlic in the olive oil for five

minutes. Add in the tomatoes, rosemary, marjoram, thyme, and chickpeas and Cooking Time: three more minutes. Add in the salt, spinach, and spaghetti squash and Cooking Time: for five more minutes while stirring constantly. Sprinkle on the chopped parsley all over the top and serve.

Nutrition:

- Calories 272
- 14 grams carbs
- 11 grams protein
- 10 grams fat

Eggplant Casserole

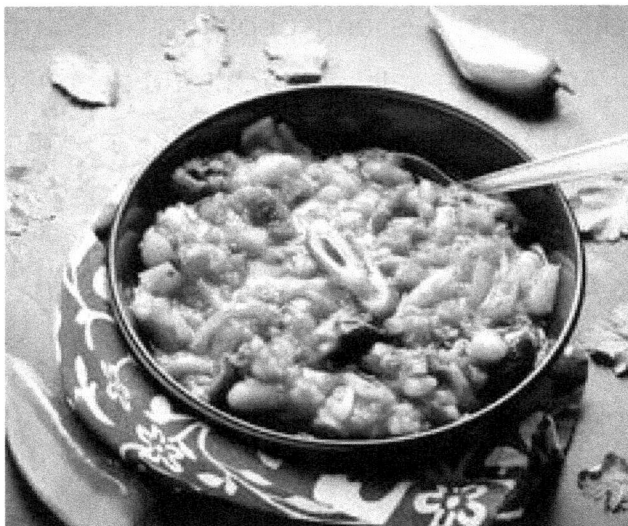

Preparation Time: 5 min

Cooking Time: 30 min

servings: 6

Ingredients:

- Eggplant, one medium
- Tomato soup, one can
- Rosemary, one teaspoon
- Salt, one half teaspoon
- Onion, chopped, one quarter cup

- Celery, one-half cup chopped fine
- Shallots, one-quarter cup chopped fine
- Olive oil, two tablespoons

Method:

Heat oven to 375. Peel the eggplant and dice it into bite-sized cubes. Drop the cubes into boiling water and Cooking Time: them for five minutes, then drain them well. Put the eggplant in a nine by nine-inch baking pan. Fry the onion, celery, and shallots in the olive oil for five minutes. Pour in the soup and cook, stirring often, for five minutes. Pour this mixture over the eggplant in the baking dish and bake for thirty minutes.

Nutrition:

- Calories 267
- 19 grams carbs
- 13 grams protein
- 9 grams fat

Butternut Squash with Mustard Vinaigrette

Preparation Time: 20 min

Cooking Time: 50 min

servings: 6

Ingredients:

- Squash, three small butternuts peeled, seeded and cut in half
- Shallots, eight, cut into wedges
- Dry mustard, one tablespoon
- Olive oil, four tablespoons
- Salt, one half teaspoon
- Turmeric, one teaspoon
- Black pepper, one teaspoon
- Balsamic vinegar, one tablespoon
- Parsley, chopped, one quarter cup

Method:

Heat oven to 375. Use a large mixing bowl to mix the shallots and the squash with the salt, pepper, turmeric, and olive oil, tossing these to mix well and coat all of the pieces. Arrange the squash and shallots on a cookie sheet and bake them for fifty minutes. While the veggies are baking make vinaigrette with the balsamic vinegar, dry mustard, and the parsley. Arrange the baked veggies on a serving dish and drizzle the vinaigrette over them and serve.

Nutrition:

- Calories 135
- 11 grams carbs
- 1 gram protein
- 10 grams fat

Mini Black Bean Pitas

Preparation Time: 1 hour 10 minutes

Cooking Time: 30 min

servings: 8

Ingredients:

- Black Beans
- Black beans, canned drained and rinsed, two cups
- Black pepper, one teaspoon
- Lemon juice, two tablespoons
- Lemon zest, one tablespoon
- Coriander, ground, three quarters teaspoon
- Cumin, ground, one teaspoon
- Garlic powder, two teaspoons
- Olive oil, one quarter cup
- Paprika, smoked, one quarter teaspoon
- Sauce
- Tomatoes, two chopped
- Dill, fresh, two tablespoons chopped
- Garlic, minced, one tablespoon

- Romaine lettuce, four leaves shred
- Lemon juice, one tablespoon
- Cucumber, one half thin sliced
- Salt, one half teaspoon
- Parsley, fresh, one quarter cup chop
- Black pepper, one teaspoon
- Red onion, one half thin sliced
- Mini pita breads, sixteen

Method:

Mix coriander, cumin, pepper, lemon juice, lemon zest, paprika, garlic powder, and olive oil and pour over the black beans in a bowl. Let this rest in the refrigerator for one hour. In another bowl, mix dill, parsley, pepper, salt, garlic, and lemon juice. Refrigerate this mixture immediately. Place the black beans with the marinade in a skillet over medium-high heat and Cooking Time: until it boils. Let this mixture simmer over low heat until the liquid is cooked off, stirring frequently. Fill the pitas with the black beans and the sauce.

Nutrition info per wrap:

Beans:

- Calories 154
- 16 grams fat
- 10 grams carbs.
- 9 grams protein

Sauce:

- Calories 300
- 5 grams fat
- 56 grams carbs
- 13 grams protein

Pasta ala Erbe

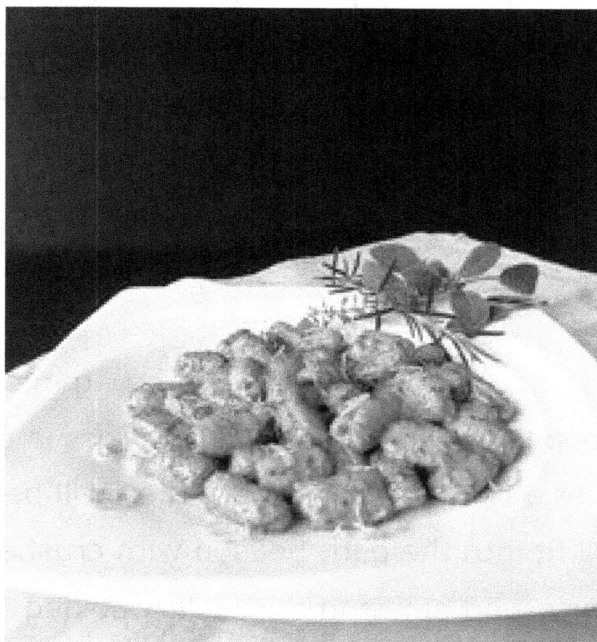

Preparation Time: 40 min

servings: 8

Ingredients:

- Whole-wheat Fettucine, one pound
- Tomato paste, two tablespoons
- Hot water, one cup
- Red pepper, crushed, one quarter teaspoon
- Rosemary, one teaspoon

- Salt, one half teaspoon
- Garlic, four cloves peeled and sliced thin
- Olive oil, six tablespoons divide
- Leafy greens, such as beet/chard/spinach, 1.5 pounds chop (no stems)

Method:

Cooking Time: the pasta per the package instructions. Cooking Time: the garlic in four tablespoons of oil for two minutes. Toss in the greens a little at a time. As they cook, they will begin to wilt and will fit into the pan. Season with crushed pepper, rosemary, and salt and stir well. Cooking Time: this mixture for about ten minutes. Blend the water into the tomato paste. Add this to skillet and simmer for fifteen minutes. Add in the cooked pasta to the skillet mix and toss well.

Nutrition info:

- Calories 355
- 14 grams fat
- 9 grams fiber
- 48 grams carbs
- 13 grams protein

Vegetarian Nachos

Preparation Time: 15 minutes

servings: 6

Ingredients:

- Oregano, dried, one tablespoon minced
- Olive oil, two tablespoons
- Hummus, one-third cup prepared
- Red onion, two tablespoons minced
- Black olives, two tablespoons chopped
- Tofu, one-half cup cut into small crumbles
- Black pepper, one half teaspoon
- Lemon juice, one tablespoon
- Grape tomatoes, one-half cup cut in quarters
- Romaine lettuce, one cup chopped
- Pita chips, whole-wheat , three cups
- Nutritional yeast, one half cup

Method:

Blend together the lemon juice, oil, pepper, and hummus in a bowl. Spread a layer of the pita chips on a platter. Use a spoon to dribble three-fourths of the hummus mix over the chips. Garnish the chips with the olives, tomatoes, red onion, and lettuce. Spoon the remainder of the hummus decoratively in the middle and garnish with the nutritional yeast and the oregano.

Nutrition info one serving:

- Calories 159
- 10 grams fat
- 2 grams fiber
- 13 grams carbs
- 4 grams proteins

Lasagna Zucchini Rolls

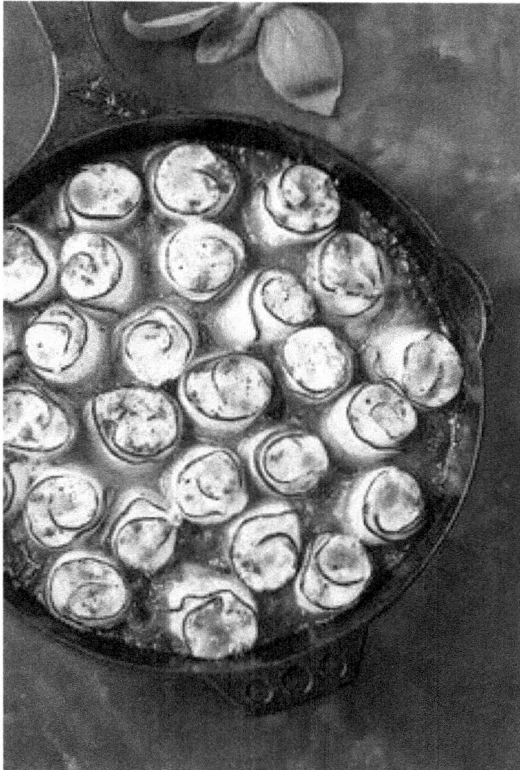

Preparation Time: 45 min

Cooking Time: 30 min

servings: 4

Ingredients:

- Zucchini, three large trimmed
- Almonds, chopped, one quarter cup
- Black pepper, one half teaspoon
- Crushed red pepper, one quarter teaspoon
- Garlic, minced, two teaspoons and two teaspoons
- Italian seasoning, one teaspoon
- Crushed tomatoes, two cups
- Salt, one-quarter teaspoon and one quarter teaspoon
- Olive oil, four tablespoons divided

Method:

Heat oven to 425. Spray oil a large cookie sheet. Cut slices from each zucchini down the length about one-quarter inch thick. Use three tablespoons of the olive oil to coat the strips and then sprinkle on one-quarter teaspoon of the salt. Bake the strips for twenty-five minutes until the zucchini strips are soft. Lower the oven temp to 350. In a bowl, mix the two teaspoons of the minced garlic, black pepper, crushed red pepper, Italian seasoning, and the tomatoes and mix well. Pour the tomato mix into a greased nine by thirteen-inch baking pan. Roll up each strip of zucchini and place it into the tomato mix in pan. Bake these for thirty minutes. Garnish with the rest of the garlic and the chopped almonds.

Nutrition info per four rolls with sauce:

- Calories 324
- 21 grams fat
- 4 grams fiber
- 19 grams carbs
- 17 grams protein

Sweet Potato and Black Bean Rice Bowl

Preparation Time: 30 min

servings: 4

Ingredients:

- Sweet chili sauce, two tablespoons
- Black beans, one fifteen ounce can drain and rinse
- Kale, fresh, four cups chopped
- Red onion, one fine chop
- Olive oil, three tablespoons
- Water, one and one half cups
- Sweet potato, two peeled and chopped into bite-sized pieces
- Celery, one-half cup chopped
- Garlic salt, one quarter teaspoon
- Turmeric, one teaspoon
- Oregano, one teaspoon
- Long grain rice, three-fourths cup uncooked

Method:

Cooking Time: the rice in water with the garlic salt for

twenty minutes. While the rice cooks put the sweet potato in the olive oil in a skillet and Cooking Time: for eight minutes, stirring often. Mix in the kale, celery, turmeric, oregano, onion, and beans and Cooking Time: for five more minutes. Stir in the chili sauce into the cooked rice and add to the potato mix; serve.

Nutrition info two cups:

- Calories 453
- 8 grams fiber
- 11 grams fat
- 10 grams protein
- 74 grams carbs

Macaroni and Cheese

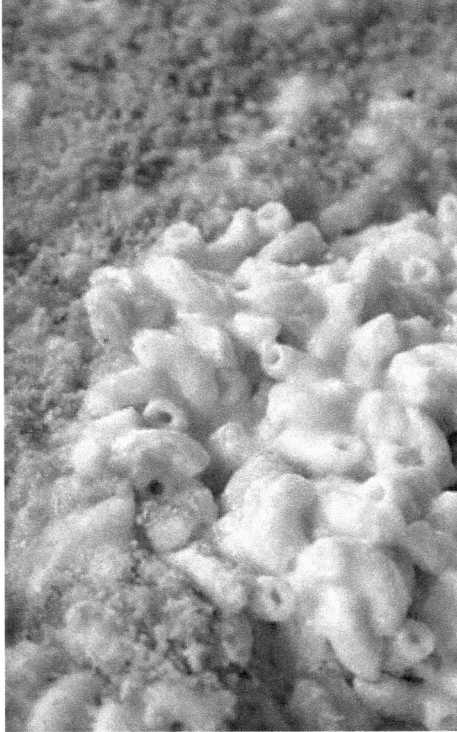

Preparation Time: 15 min

Cooking Time: 25 min

servings: 4

Ingredients:

- Elbow macaroni, whole-grain , eight ounces
- Apple cider vinegar, two teaspoons

- Water, one cup (more if needed)
- Red pepper, flakes, one eighth teaspoon
- Salt, one half teaspoon
- Dry mustard powder, one half teaspoon
- Onion powder, one half teaspoon
- Garlic powder, one half teaspoon
- Garlic, minced, two tablespoons
- Russet potato, peeled and grated, one cup (about two small potatoes)
- Onion, yellow, chopped, one cup
- Avocado oil, two tablespoons
- Broccoli, one head with florets cut into bite-sized pieces
- Nutritional yeast, one quarter cup

Method:

Cooking Time: the elbow pasta according to the directions on the package. When the pasta is almost done (with two or three minutes left), stir in the broccoli with the pasta. Drain the broccoli past mix and place it in a large bowl. During the time the pasta is cooking warm the olive oil in a saucepan over medium-high heat and Cooking Time: the salt and the onion for about five minutes. Stir in the onion powder, grated potato, garlic powder, mustard powder, and salt, garlic, and red pepper flakes. Mix this well and let it cooks for two minutes so the flavors will mix. Pour in the water and mix well. Continue stirring frequently while this mixture cooks for about eight to ten minutes until the potatoes are tender. Pour this mixture carefully into a blender with the vinegar and the nutritional yeast and blend carefully until it is smooth and creamy. Pour this mix over the past in the large bowl, mix well, and serve.

Nutrition:

- Calories 506
- 21.7 grams fat
- 66.5 grams carbs
- 8.7 grams fiber
- 18.3 grams protein

Avocado, Kale, and Black Bean Bowl

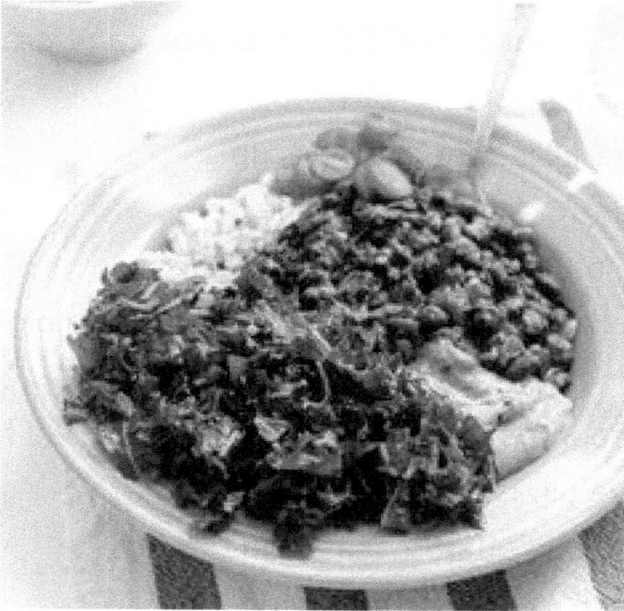

Preparation Time: 20 min

Cooking Time: 30 min

servings: 4

Ingredients:

- Kale, one bunch with ribs removed and chopped into bite-sized pieces
- Cherry tomatoes, cut in half, one half cup
- Cayenne pepper, one quarter teaspoon

- Chili powder, one quarter teaspoon
- Garlic, minced, two tablespoons
- Shallot, one chopped finely
- Black beans, two fifteen ounce cans drained and rinsed
- Lime juice, one quarter cup
- Cilantro, chopped, one half cup
- Salsa Verde, mild, one half cup
- Avocado, one, peeled, pitted, cut into big chunks
- Cumin, one half teaspoon
- Jalapeno, one half, seeded and chopped finely
- Olive oil, two tablespoons
- Salt, one quarter teaspoon
- Brown rice, one cup rinsed

Method:

Cooking Time: the rice per the package instructions and then let it rest for fifteen minutes and then salt the rice and fluff it with a fork. While the rice is cooking, make the kale salad by blending together the cumin, salt, olive oil, jalapeno, and the lime juice and then put in the chopped kale. In another bowl, mix together well the cilantro, lime juice, Salsa Verde, and the chunks of the avocado. Place the beans in a saucepan and warm them over low heat in one tablespoon of olive oil. Mix in the shallot and the garlic and Cooking Time: for three minutes, then stir in the chili powder and cayenne pepper. Cooking Time: for seven to ten minutes. For serving, add the kale salad with the rice and the bean mixture to bowls and add in some of the Salsa Verde avocado. Toss chopped cherry tomatoes on top for garnish.

Nutrition:

- Calories 424
- 12 grams fat
- 57 grams carbs
- 12 grams fiber
- 24 grams protein

www.ingramcontent.com/pod-product-compliance
Lightning Source LLC
Chambersburg PA
CBHW070722030426
42336CB00013B/1894